I0440935

101 ways to exercise without noticing.

Marianne Duvall.

ISBN-13: 978-1484137123

ISBN-10: 1484137124

Contents

Introduction

Exercise.

We should all do more of it! And the very word 'exercise' conjures up a mental picture of training for a marathon or pounding the treadmill in a gym full of ultra-fit people looking at you sweating.

Ugh! It's enough to make you curl up on the sofa with a bag of crisps.

But what is exercise?

Basically it's movement. And moving more than you would normally move, means that you are getting more exercise. This book is all about giving you some ideas of how you can increase your activity in normal daily life.

So forget the gym membership, which most people do after the first couple of weeks anyway, even though they keep exercising their bank accounts by paying for it each month.

Forget the early morning run, the sweaty tracksuit and running shoes. Learn how to exercise without noticing.

Although some of us hate doing it and for others exercise is incredibly difficult, it is still vitally important for good health. So being able to find a way of increasing the amount of exercise in our daily life easily is important.

Exercise and activity is not only involved in weight loss, it affects how well our entire body functions. The heart rate, metabolism and blood pressure are all affected by the amount of activity in our daily lives.

Many people just see exercise as a way of burning calories, but it actually improves your entire metabolism so that even when you're not active you still burn more calories than you would otherwise have done.

Improving your level of activity will help protect you from heart disease, type2 diabetes, osteoporosis and many other chronic diseases. It will also make you feel better. Increased activity, especially something like a walk in the park, can lift your mood and even help with problems of depression or anxiety.

This list of *101 ways to exercise without noticing*, is intended to give you some ideas rather than being an exhaustive list or a plan you should follow from beginning to end. Dip into it and pick the ideas that work for you, adapting them to your lifestyle, adding some of your own as you go along.

It doesn't take long before the added activity begins to make a real difference to how you feel and then it becomes easier to add even more activity, creating a virtuous circle that will lead to greater fitness without you really noticing.

Walking and exercise

Walking is one of the best and easiest ways to get more movement and therefore more exercise and activity into your life. I don't mean a ten mile hike or regular power walking, I mean the ordinary walking that we do – just more of it.

The one piece of exercise equipment that you should invest in is a step counter, also called a pedometer.

You can get some very fancy ones that measure how many calories you use, how far you have walked, even if you climb stairs. They can monitor your pulse, help you set goals and download all the information to your computer, but all you really need is a basic but accurate pedometer that counts how many steps you take during the day.

The more steps you do, the more you are exercising and it is very encouraging to see the total mount up. Many experts say that you should do 10,000 steps a day, but don't get discouraged by that. Make a note of how many steps you are doing when you start and every increase you can make on that is an improvement. So even when you change from 500 to 1000 steps a day, you've doubled your walking activity.

Keep a record so you can see the totals increase, it's very motivating to see that you are actually making a difference as the days and weeks go on, and that it's all happening without you really noticing.

And the great thing is, the more you do the more you can do, it really does work one step at a time.

The obvious first step is to actually increase the number of steps you do in a day. Ideally you will walk fast enough to get slightly out of breath, the type of out of breath that will allow you to still carry on a conversation with someone but where you would struggle to sing. Of course many of us would struggle to sing at the best of times!

There are plenty of opportunities to increase the level of exercise by small amounts as we go through normal daily life, opportunities that we often don't really think about, and as they say, every little helps.

1: If you drive to work or to the shops, get into the habit of parking a little bit further away than you would normally do. Stop looking for a parking place as close to the doors as possible and choose a place halfway down the car park. As you get more used to this you can park further and further away.

2: If you can, park downhill or uphill from where you are going. Even a short walk is more effective combined with a hill.

3: If you take the bus, get off one stop earlier than normal or walk to the next bus stop instead of the one you normally use. As this gets easier, get off two stops early. Eventually for shorter journeys you'll get into the habit of not using the bus at all.

4: At the supermarket carry a basket rather than using a small trolley, you'll be getting some weight training along with getting your vegetables. It has the added benefit of making you think about each item that you put in the basket rather than just throwing it into a trolley. After all, each extra item adds to the weight you are carrying on your arm.

5: Be less efficient in the supermarket. Walk up and down every aisle rather than missing out the ones you don't need. You can double or triple the number of steps you take in this way.

6: You can even criss-cross the store, deliberately going to the further aisle first and then backwards and forwards across the store filling your basket, rather than efficiently going to the next, closest point each time. It might mean your shopping takes a few minutes longer but it's worth it for the extra steps you'll be taking.

7: Go and collect your morning paper from the newsagent, rather than having it delivered. Walk to the shop, of course! It's a good way of starting your day by getting your body moving.

8: If you have a choice of shops within walking distance, choose the one further away.

9: If you have a dog, treat it to a longer walk. Good for both of you. If you don't have a dog of your own, can you walk a friend's or neighbour's dog?

10: Learn to embrace the idea that there's no such thing as bad weather, just the wrong clothing. It's far too easy to take the car a short distance because it's wet or cold. Wrap up properly and walk.

11: When you do walk, pick up the pace a bit. Stride rather than stroll. You can increase your speed gradually, but it is much better for you if you stride out. You will get slightly breathless which is better exercise.

12: If you have shops close by, walk to them and buy smaller amounts so that you can carry them by hand rather than needing transport.

13: Buy smaller amounts so that you have to walk to the shops more often.

14: Use the stairs rather than lift. It sounds obvious but you don't just have to think it means only going upstairs. Walking downstairs is also good exercise but much easier to start with. And you don't have to start with the whole distance, use the stairs for a floor or two and the lift for the rest.

15: If you take the lift from a high floor, start by getting out a floor early and walking down the rest of the way

16: As you get used to it, walk down more flights of stairs.

17: Then you can start getting out a floor early and walking up a flight of stairs.

18: Get into the habit of looking for the stairs rather than the lift or escalator. It's amazing how quickly this will become a habit.

19: If you do find yourself using the escalator, walk up it rather than just standing still and letting it carry you. Only do this on the up escalator. It can be dangerous to do it on a downward escalator. And make sure you never run on an escalator, safety is very important.

20: Try leaving things upstairs, then you will have to go up and get them rather than being organised and bringing everything down at once. For instance when you're going out make sure that you're going to have to go back upstairs to the wardrobe to get your coat.

Housework and exercise

Housework is a great form of everyday exercise and you also have the benefit of having a spotless, tidy home! It's certainly a lot cheaper than gym membership.

Housework is something that we all have to do and sometimes it's very difficult to fit in the time for it, but if you start to think of it as exercise rather than having to make separate time for exercise as well as the housework, you can start to save time as well as money.

21: Rather than using the washing machine or dry cleaners all the time, try washing some of your clothes by hand, it can be quite a physical task. As a bonus, your delicate clothes of lace, cashmere or silk will be kept in better condition

22: Get into the habit of ironing everything that you can, not only a small selection of smart work clothes! That means the sheets, towels, pillowcases and casual clothes, the items that you would normally leave to just drip dry. Ironing is a great exercise for the upper body and one of the jobs that you stand to do. Standing is much better than sitting. You should try to stand regularly throughout the day.

23: If you can, hang washing outside on the line rather than using a tumble dryer. Hanging washing on a line involves lots of stretching and bending.

24: Clean your own windows rather than paying a window cleaner to do it for you. At least do the downstairs windows yourself. Again, lots of stretching and bending.

25: Wash your car by hand rather than taking it to a carwash. Washing a car properly can be a surprisingly physical job, plenty more stretching and bending.

26: Once you finish washing and drying it properly, treat your car to a good polish with a coat of wax. Again, lots of stretching and bending, a good full body workout and you'll be protecting the paintwork of your car at the same time.

27: Clean the inside of your car rather than paying for a valet service and make sure that you get into all the corners. This involves lots of movement. Twisting, stretching, reaching into the far corners of the vehicle - it's another full body workout when you do it properly.

28: Make the bed properly every morning rather than just shaking the duvet. If you don't have time in the morning leave the bed to air and make it in the evening. Straightening sheets, shaking up the duvet, punching the pillows and putting it all back together again will add quite a bit of exercise to your daily list.

29: Use the vacuum cleaner every day, it involves lots of movement, twisting and stretching.

30: Vacuum the stairs. This involves plenty of movement because it can be quite an awkward job and one you tend to leave, but it is great exercise. If you're feeling really active you can use dustpan and brush instead!

31: And for more stretching and moving, try high dusting on a regular basis. Put some music on while you doing it, this makes it much more fun and it's far more practical than putting on a dance exercise DVD. You know, one of those things that tend to gather dust in the corner of the room!

32: In fact any dusting and polishing involves movement. Reaching stretching, moving things and putting them back - so get into the habit of taking out the duster and polish regularly.

33: If you have wooden furniture, start treating it to a regular wax polish. It's great for the furniture, it will keep it in tiptop condition and make it last so much longer. And if you really work hard at it, it will even achieve that magical goal of exercise, you will be breathless!

34: Clean down the back of the furniture. The places most people forget. But shifting all those cushions, using the vacuum or pan and brush and putting all the cushions back in place again is quite a bit of exercise. You might even find some coins down there.

The Kitchen and exercise

The kitchen can make a wonderful home gym, especially if you put away the modern effort saving gadgets.

There are so many opportunities for good physical movement, the type that can help build up your muscles, especially your upper body muscle.

It also has the benefit of making you take more notice of the food you are eating, getting you more in touch with the food you are preparing rather than just tearing open convenience food.

35: Don't buy prepared packs of vegetables, buy the actual vegetables and prepare them yourself. Not only will you save money on your groceries, but cleaning, peeling and chopping vegetables is great exercise.

36: Put your electric mixer in the cupboard when making a cake and stir that mix yourself! Very satisfying.

37: Store items that you use most often in a high cupboard where you will have to stretch to get them.

38: When the high cupboards are full, put the rest of your regular items in a low cupboard, which will add bending to your exercise workout.

39: Remember, in all different ways, convenience is the enemy of exercise. We have surrounded ourselves with gadgets and tools whose very purpose is to make life easier and less physical. It's time to put some of these away.

40: When you're going to make a cappuccino or frothy chocolate, whisk it by hand rather than gadget. Alternate your hands as you're whisking so that both arms get stronger. You would be amazed how difficult using a whisk is at first, in fact it can be horrifying to discover just how unfit you are! But it's also surprising and gratifying how quickly your arm strength will improve.

41: Clean the inside of your oven regularly. This is quite a physical job with a lot of awkward stretching and reaching. And if you have a freestanding cooker rather than the built-in eyelevel oven, you will also have to kneel down or squat to do it, which involves exercising your thigh muscles as well.

42: When you have to open any tins or cans, use an old-fashioned tin opener rather than an electric model.

43: Squeeze orange, grapefruit or lemon juice yourself on a hand press rather than working with an electric gadget.

44: Use hand grinders for your salt and pepper rather than the fancy powered designs. It might not take long, but as they say every little helps.

45: Use a shaker when making your salad dressing - a great little workout - you can get surprisingly breathless mixing up the good salad dressing! It's good cardiovascular exercise and will help you build up some arm muscles.

46: Use a hand blender when making a milkshake or a smoothie, you might have to mush up the fruit by hand first for a smoothie, but that makes it an even better workout.

47: Wash up by hand rather than using a dishwasher, especially on dirty pots and pans.

48: And then dry them with a tea towel, rather than just leaving them on the drainer.

49: When you're at the supermarket avoid buying bags of grated cheese, buy blocks of cheese instead and grate it yourself.

50: Buy unsliced bread and learn to love your bread knife. It also means everyone in the family can have bread the thickness that they prefer. Even better if you decide to make your own bread – by hand not in a bread machine of course, you'll be surprised how much irritation you can get rid of with a good bit of bread kneading!

51: In general, if you need ingredients sliced, grated, minced or diced, buy the raw ingredients and use hand powered tools to do the job. That means knives, graters, grinders and the chopping block – and of course, that good old fashioned elbow grease!

Gardening and exercise

The garden is a wonderful source of free exercise, and you'll be getting plenty of healthy fresh air and building up your vitamin D while you do it.

You can use your garden or allotment to improve your health by growing some of your own fresh fruit and vegetables as well. Food that is slow grown rather than forced and organic rather than full of chemicals tastes better and is better for your health, full of the vitamins and minerals that we need.

Vitamins D deficiency is becoming a problem in our modern society because we are simply not spending enough time outside in the sunshine and our bodies create vitamin D through the interaction of natural sunlight on the skin.

So a good session in the garden is good for the body in all sorts of ways.

52: Do yourself and your lawn a favour, mow it regularly. If you can, you could invest in an old-fashioned hand mower. Much more exercise, it will cut your electricity bill, and it's much more environmentally friendly.

53: Once you've cut the grass, rake your lawn. It's great for creating a healthy lawn, getting rid of moss and wonderful cardiovascular exercise, as well as great for your core muscles.

54: Hoe the flower and vegetable beds regularly, it will keep the weeds at bay and make your flower or vegetable beds look great. And again wonderful stretching, twisting and cardiovascular exercise.

55: Trim the lawn edges. It makes the garden neat and tidy and is very good exercise for the upper body.

56: Dig your beds over before you plant in the spring and dig in some good organic fertiliser and compost.

57: Use shears rather than an electric trimmer on your hedges. This can be wonderful exercise, lots of stretching and reaching makes it a wonderful workout for the upper body, it's also a good balancing exercise. And if your hedges are higher, it's good exercise for the thighs and calves. In fact, it's such good exercise that you'll probably need to soak in the bath afterwards!

58: Wash your greenhouse out if you have one, cleaning all the windows and getting into all the corners and edges.

59: Use a small hand trowel and fork on your beds. You have to kneel down to get to them and then stretch around the bed as you work.

60: When you're pruning shrubs, cut the branches into smaller pieces. More cuts, more exercise and it takes up less space in your rubbish bin or compost heap.

61: If you have room in your garden for a compost heap, have one and turn it regularly. It's great for you, for your garden, for the environment and a great source of exercise for you.

62: Clean your patio or decking with a brush and bucket of water rather than using a power washer.

63: Paint any fences or sheds you have with a brush rather than a paint sprayer. Lots of stretching and bending.

64: Clean any wooden furniture in your garden in the spring, scrubbing off any moss and dirt that it has gathered over the year. Then treat it to a coat of oil to protect it and make it look good. Remember to let it dry before collapsing for a rest!

65: Instead of trimming the hedge once a year, do it twice a year. Good for the hedge, good for you.

Children and exercise

Having small children can be one of the greatest forms of exercise you'll ever find, as well as being the one time in your life when you really need to be as fit as you can be.

Children need, in fact demand attention and it's so much better for you and them if they have an active childhood and you are active with them.

You will have more energy to deal with them if you are fitter yourself and you will be instilling the right attitudes for them to go on and have a fit and healthy life themselves.

Build activity into every day that you can, even if it's only for short bursts during the week and then plan more fun time at the weekends. Avoid the danger of the TV and games consuls, they're great fun but they can take over a child's life and you need to show them that there is much more to life.

As another bonus, running round in the park, playing cricket or football, skating or cycling will burn up their excess energy in a way that no computer game will!

66: Use a baby carrier as much as you can, instead of a pram or buggy, you'll find it builds up great arm muscles. Make sure that you swap arms regularly so that your muscles are even and you'll end up with great biceps.

67: When you go to the playpark, push those swings hard. Your kids will love it!

68: Play with your kids. Youngsters are full of energy and love to play. So get involved rather than just sitting on the sidelines watching.

69: Sometimes, dealing with young children can feel a bit like a wrestling match. Rather than getting annoyed with them, learn to embrace and enjoy it, this is a great fun form of exercise.

70: Invest in a trampoline for your children if you have enough space and use it yourself as well. It's fun!

71: Build physical activity into every day you spend with your children, whether it's going for a walk, playing in the park or kicking a ball round in the back garden. It's wonderful training for children, showing them how to have an active life rather than just sitting in front of the TV. And it's fantastic exercise for you.

Work and exercise

Most of us spend a great deal of time at work. So it's important to try and include some exercise into these 40 hours a week. Some jobs make this easy, if you deliver the mail you'll be walking miles every day but if you work in an office or behind a counter it can be a little more difficult.

Finding some simple ways to include physical movement into your day will make you feel better, keep you more alert and make the day less mentally tiring.

72: Spend as much time standing at work as you can. Many jobs involve a lot of sitting, but it's much better if you can intersperse this with periods of standing. So stand whenever you have the opportunity rather than looking for the nearest seat. For instance, when you're having a conversation, when you're at the photocopier or even when you're on the telephone.

73: If you have the opportunity, go out during your lunch break. You might be able to go for a short walk around the local area or it might just be a walk to the canteen or the local sandwich shop, but at least you are moving, adding some steps to your total daily tally. If you have the chance to go outside, do take the opportunity rather than staying inside sitting at your desk.

74: When something needs moving or collecting at work, don't wait for somebody else to do it, go and do it yourself.

75: When you are sitting in a chair when working, take every opportunity you have to stretch or move. You can easily do leg stretches sitting at a desk. Lift one leg until it is parallel with the floor, hold it for a few seconds, flexing your foot so that your toes point out, and then point to the ceiling. Lower your leg slowly and repeat with the other leg.

76: Stretch your arms above your head as if you're reaching for a very high shelf. Not only is this good exercise, it will ease tension in your shoulders and reduce back ache and headaches.

77: If you work in a large building, try to take the long way round when you have to go anywhere, using stairs rather than the lift whenever possible.

78: If you do have a job which involves a lot of sitting, take the opportunity to stand up and move whenever possible.

79: If you can, store things on high shelves or in low cupboards so that you have to bend and stretch to get the things you need every day.

80: If you have to carry things at work, gradually increase your load rather than taking small amounts, this is a good way of increasing your strength.

81: On the other hand, you could keep your load small so that you have to make more journeys and increase the amount of steps you do each day.

82: When you need to visit the bathroom at work, choose one that's further away, especially if you can go to a bathroom on another floor - using the stairs to get there of course.

83: When you need to talk to a colleague in another part of the building don't just e-mail or pick up the phone, go and see them.

84: If you do work at a desk, get into the habit of standing up and walking around the office for a few minutes every hour. It could simply be a walk to the water cooler, which would improve your hydration as well as your exercise.

Leisure and exercise

Although you might not want to spend your leisure time and weekends at the gym or running round the track, there are still ways of increasing your level of activity while relaxing.

Not only will you benefit from getting more exercise, you can also get fresh air and a chance to spend more time with your friends and family.

Fresh air, exercise and fun with friends - a great mix for your mental and emotional wellbeing as well as your physical health.

85: Dust off the bicycle that is lurking at the back of the shed. Give it a good clean, check that everything is in working order – a great piece of exercise in itself.

86: Pump up the tires if they need it, lubricate the exposed moving parts such as the chain or the gear mechanisms, although make sure you don't get any on the wheel rims or the brake blocks. If it's a while since you have used your bike you should give it a full service to make sure that it is safe. If you need to, get it checked professionally to make sure that everything is right on it.

87: Now that your bike is safe again, go out for a ride at the weekend. Of course, you can also choose to use your bike rather than the car for everyday transport or at least a few times a week.

88: If you don't want to go for a bike ride, go for a nice long walk in the countryside at the weekend. If you can't get to the countryside, most of us live close to a park.

89: When you're going out with a group of friends or family, choose something active like the bowling alley rather than the cinema. Great fun, more interactive, and certainly more active for all of you.

90: Rather than just going to the local pub, choose somewhere with music where you can dance and move.

91: Go to a car boot sale where you can walk miles up and down and around the field. Don't go logically up and down the aisles, take the long way round.

92: If you like visiting stately homes don't miss out the gardens. Take long walks to the furthest ends of the grounds.

93: Take up an active new hobby, such as swimming, surfing, canoeing, mountain biking, rock climbing, tennis or anything else you've always wanted to try. Exercise never feels like exercise when you're having fun.

94: Get involved with local community activities such as coaching the local sports team, working with the local gardening project or helping decorate homes for those who can't manage it themselves.

DIY and exercise

Although it is not an everyday activity for most of us, DIY can be an excellent form of exercise.

So there's no need to put off decorating the house with the excuse that you have to go down the gym!

And of course the more time and effort you put in to it, the better the finished work should be and the more exercise you will have had.

95: Do your own painting and decorating and make sure that you do the preparation work as well, lots of bending and stretching. Sanding is an excellent upper body and cardiovascular workout – done with a sanding block of course, not an electric sander! Then there's all carrying and shifting and every type of movement you can think of.

96: When you're painting the woodwork on the outside of your house, make sure that you prepare it properly. Rub it down first, removing any old flaking paintwork and preparing a smooth surface before you start the new paint. You can make it an even more professional job by using masking tape around the glass to make sure you don't paint the window, as well as the window frame. More reaching and stretching!

97: When you are building flat pack furniture or putting up new shelves, put the power tools away and use good old-fashioned hand tools and muscle power. Dig out your hand saws, chisels, hand planes and sanding blocks rather than all those wonderful enticing power tools!

Posture and exercise

There are also some simple changes you can make to the way you move as you go about your everyday life that will make your muscles work harder and help you burn a few extra calories.

They may feel strange at first, but once you get used to them they'll become second nature and you'll be making your body work more efficiently, improving your muscle tone and your metabolism.

98: Bend at the knees and squat when you want to pick something up off the floor, it will exercise your thigh muscles. Try to hold the squat for a few seconds before standing up slowly. If plies and demi-plies are good enough for ballet dancers, they are good enough for the rest of us!

99: Get into the habit of pulling your stomach in as you stand or sit, even as you drive. It's great exercise for the stomach muscles and will help build your core strength.

100: It might look strange, but when you can, take the opportunity to stand on one leg and improve your balance. You could do it while standing at the sink washing up or washing your hands.

101: Try and think about your posture and ways of improving it as often as you can. Stand straight, put your shoulders back and sit up straight. All of these things will improve the way you hold your body. It will give your internal organs the space they need to function properly and will have a generally improving affect on your health.

Once you start thinking of the ways that you can increase your activity during the day you will find more and more ways of doing it that will fit in with your lifestyle and timetable.

Anything that increases the amount of movement you make and the amount of activity that you take during the day will improve your level of exercise and therefore your level of fitness.

As time goes by, try to make the exercise more strenuous. For instance walk faster, carry heavier weights, take the stairs two at a time or run up the stairs rather than walking.

As you add more activity into your daily life you'll begin to feel better and be able to do more physical things more easily.

You'll find that you don't get breathless when doing simple tasks, you won't ache when you have to walk instead of take the car, you won't worry when you find that the lift is out of order and you have to use the stairs.

You'll feel better, feel fitter, breathe easier and find yourself adding more and more activity to your life without ever really noticing.

About the Author

Marianne Duvall's passion in life is showing people how to make it easy to live a healthier life through nutrition and fitness – making small changes in everyday life that can make big changes in health and wellbeing.

She has studied how to rebalance modern life to allow space for good nutrition and activity as part of everyday life rather than an expensive and time consuming extra.

She believes that healthy living should be how we live, part of everyday life rather than an afterthought. Something so natural that we don't even think about it, we just do it.

She has developed her ideas over the years working with those living with chronic illnesses such as M.E./CFS, fibromyalgia or diabetes, developing plans that help people live successfully with these illnesses.

Her motto is 'Live Life'